GW01112120

Lynne Robinson is a leading Pilates specialist, whose best-selling first book with Gordon Thomson, *Body Control – The Pilates Way*, has won wide acclaim. Widely featured on TV and in magazines for her work, she is also co-author with Helge Fisher of *Mind-Body Workout*, and is presenter of Telstar's top-selling *Body Control* video, and the new *Pilates Weekly Workout*.

Gordon Thompson, formerly of the Ballet Rambert and London Contemporary Dance, runs the prestigious Body Control Pilates Studio in London's South Kensington. He is co-author of the original *Body Control – The Pilates Way*.

Helge Fisher is qualified in anatomy, physiology and holistic massage, and is an Alexander Technique teacher. The co-author with Lynne Robinson of *Mind-Body Workout*, she has been teaching Body Control Pilates for over ten years.

Advice to the Reader

Before following any of the exercise advice contained in this book it is recommended that you consult your doctor if you suffer from any health problems or special conditions or are in any doubt as to its suitability.

Off to Sleep

Lynne Robinson, Gordon Thomson & Helge Fisher

PAN BOOKS

First published 1999 by Pan Books

an imprint of Macmillan Publishers Limited
25 Eccleston Place, London SW1W 9NF
and Basingstoke

Associated companies throughout the world

ISBN 0 330 37330 7

Copyright © Lynne Robinson, Gordon Thomson and Helge Fisher

The right of Lynne Robinson, Gordon Thomson and Helge Fisher
to be identified as the authors of this work has been asserted by them
in accordance with the Copyright, Designs and Patents Act 1988.

All rights reserved. No part of this publication may be
reproduced, stored in or introduced into a retrieval system, or
transmitted, in any form, or by any means (electronic, mechanical,
photocopying, recording or otherwise) without the prior written
permission of the publisher. Any person who does any unauthorized
act in relation to this publication may be liable to criminal
prosecution and civil claims for damages.

9 8 7 6 5 4 3 2 1

A CIP catalogue record for this book is available from the British Library.

Text design by Neil Lang
Printed and bound in Belgium

This book is sold subject to the condition that it shall not,
by way of trade or otherwise, be lent, re-sold, hired out,
or otherwise circulated without the publisher's prior consent
in any form of binding or cover other than that in which
it is published and without a similar condition including this
condition being imposed on the subsequent purchaser.

Contents

Introduction 6
The Eight Principles of the Pilates Method 7
Before You Begin 8
Checking Your Alignment 9
The Position of the Pelvis and Spine 10
Breathing the Pilates Way 12
Creating a Strong Centre 14

The Exercises

Static Hamstring Stretches 16
Side Rolls 20
Adductor Openings 24
Shoulder Circles 26
Pelvic Roll Backs 28
The Mexican Wave 32
Single Heel Kicks 34
The Big Pillow Squeeze 38
The Rest Position 40
Circle of Chalk 42
Tense and Release 46

Introduction

At the end of a hard day, all you are probably thinking about is collapsing into bed. Being tired, however, does not necessarily ensure a good night's rest. To sleep well, your mind needs to be calm, your body balanced.

The following exercises will prepare both mind and body for a sound sleep. They are designed to correct any muscle imbalances acquired during the day, realigning the body and bringing it back into its correct postural alignment. They will help to prevent you stiffening up overnight.

As you focus on the movements of your body, your mind will clear, you will feel relaxed. When you become more familiar with the exercises, they can become part of your bedtime routine, so helping you to feel more settled.

The Eight Principles of the Pilates Method

The exercises in this book have their origins in the work of Joseph Pilates (1880–1967). A well-proven method in existence for over seventy-five years, they also incorporate the latest techniques in both mental and physical training, offering complete body conditioning.

The programme targets the key postural muscles, building strength from within by stabilizing the torso. The body is gently realigned and reshaped, the muscles balanced, so that the whole body moves efficiently. By bringing together body and mind and heightening body awareness, Pilates literally teaches you to be in control of your body, allowing you to handle stress more effectively and achieve relaxation more easily.

All the exercises are built around the following Eight Principles:

Relaxation	**Co-ordination**
Concentration	**Centring**
Alignment	**Flowing movements**
Breathing	**Stamina**

Before You Begin

▷ All exercises should be done on a padded mat.
▷ Wear something warm and comfortable, allowing free movement.
▷ Barefoot is best, socks otherwise.
▷ You may need: a firm flat pillow or folded towel, a larger pillow, a long scarf and a tennis ball.

Please do not exercise if:

▷ You are feeling unwell
▷ You have just eaten a heavy meal
▷ You have a bad hangover or have been drinking alcohol
▷ You have taken painkillers, as it will mask any warning pains

If you are undergoing medical treatment, are pregnant or injured, please consult your medical practitioner. It is always advisable to consult your doctor before you take up a new exercise regime.

Checking Your Alignment

Always take a moment to check that your body is correctly aligned before you start an exercise. Here is a checklist to help:

- Is my pelvis in neutral? See page 10.
- Is my spine lengthened, but still with its natural curves? Think of the top of the head lengthening away from the tailbone.
- Where are my shoulders? Hopefully not up around your ears! Keep the shoulder blades down into your back, a nice big gap between the ears and the shoulders.
- Is my neck tense? Keep the neck released and soft, the back of the neck stays long.
- Where are my feet? Don't forget them, for if they are misplaced it will affect your knees, hips and back. Usually, they should be hip-width apart, in parallel. Watch that they do not roll in or out!

The Position of the Pelvis and Spine

If you exercise with the pelvis and the spine misplaced you run the risk of creating muscle imbalances and stressing the spine itself. You should aim to have your pelvis and spine in their natural, neutral positions.

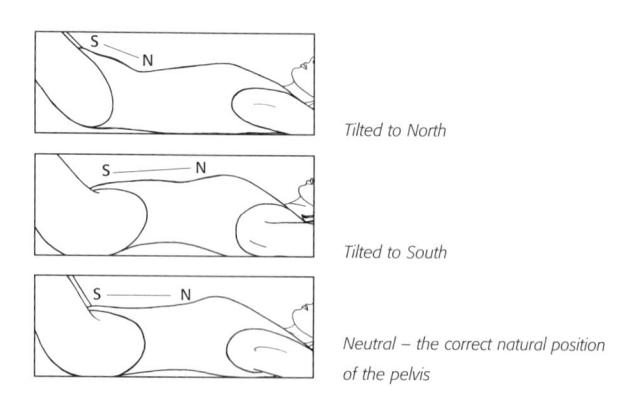

Tilted to North

Tilted to South

Neutral – the correct natural position of the pelvis

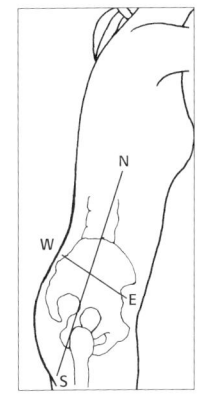

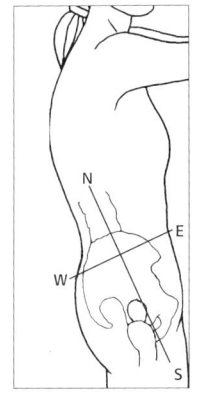

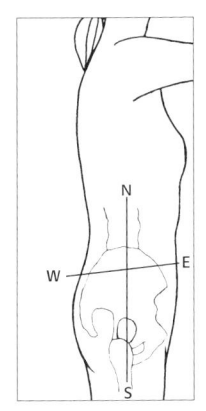

Wrong   *Wrong*   *Right*

Breathing the Pilates Way

In Pilates we use lateral, thoracic breathing for all exercises. This entails breathing into the lower ribcage and back to make maximum use of lung capacity. The increased oxygen intake replenishes the body and the action itself creates greater flexibility in the upper body. It also works the abdominals.

To learn lateral breathing you may sit, stand or kneel, your pelvis in neutral, the spine lengthened.

Wrap a scarf around your ribcage, cross the ends over in the front and pull a little on them to feel where you are working. The idea is to breathe into the scarf, directing the breath into your sides and back, but keeping the shoulders down and relaxed, and the neck calm.

The ribs expand as you inhale, close down as you exhale.

Repeat six times but do not over-breathe or you may feel dizzy.

Breathe softly in a relaxed way.

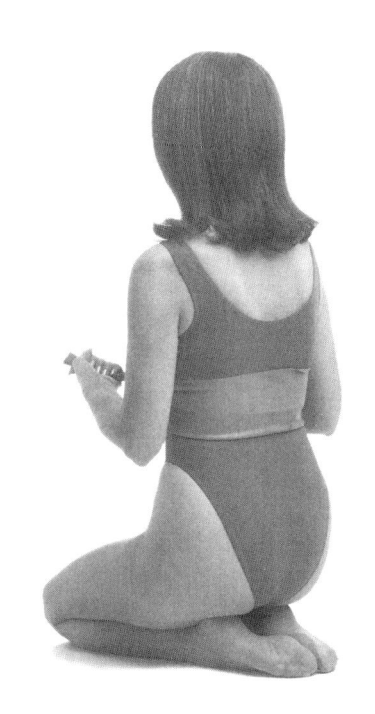

*Breathe in wide and
   full to prepare for
   movement
Breathe out as you move
Breathe in to recover*

Creating a Strong Centre

Nearly all Pilates exercises involve engaging the deep postural muscles to protect the spine as you exercise. This is called 'stabilizing' or 'centring' and creates a 'girdle of strength' from which to move.

To find these deep muscles, adopt the Starting Position opposite:

▷ Breathe in to prepare and lengthen through the spine.
▷ Breathe out and engage the muscles of your pelvic floor (as if you are trying not to pass water) and hollow your lower abdominals back to your spine. Do not move the pelvis or spine.
▷ Breathe in and release.

Think of it as an internal zip which begins underneath and zips up and in to hold your lower abdominal contents in place, just like zipping up your trousers.'**Zip up and hollow**'.

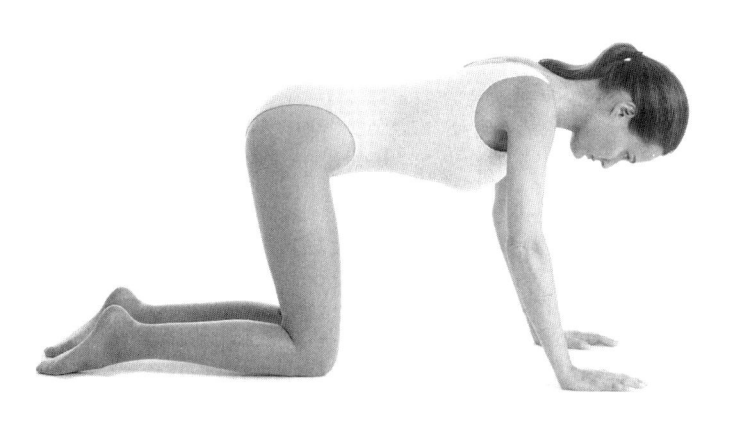

Come onto all fours, hands beneath shoulders, knees beneath your hips. Look straight down at the floor, the back of the neck stays long, the spine maintains its natural neutral curve.

Static Hamstring Stretches

Starting Position
Sit on the floor with your legs out in front of you, your pelvis square. Bend the left knee and place the sole of the foot on the inside of the right knee. Keep your right leg straight, the knee facing to the ceiling, the foot relaxed.

Action
▷ Breathe in to prepare and lengthen up through the spine.
▷ Breathe out, **zip up the pelvic floor and hollow navel to spine**, lift up and out of your pelvis and over an imaginary beach ball.

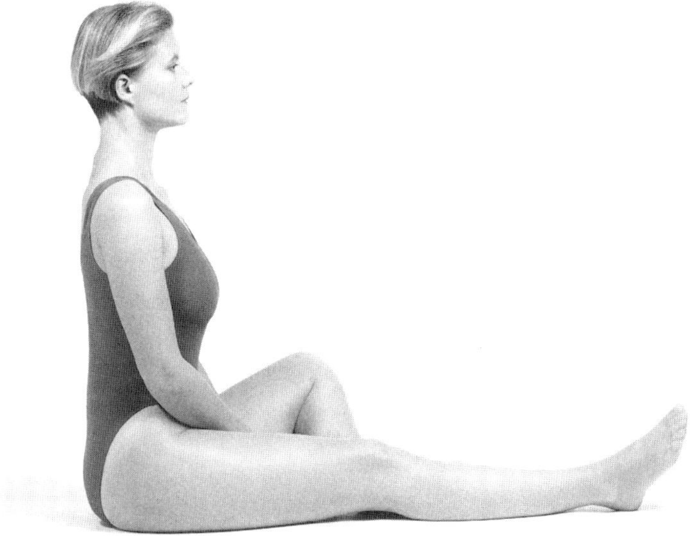

Static Hamstring Stretches (continued)

▷ Take twelve slow breaths, breathing deeply into your sides and the back of your ribcage, relaxing into the position. Keep your shoulders down into your back, your neck long and the top of your head lengthening away towards

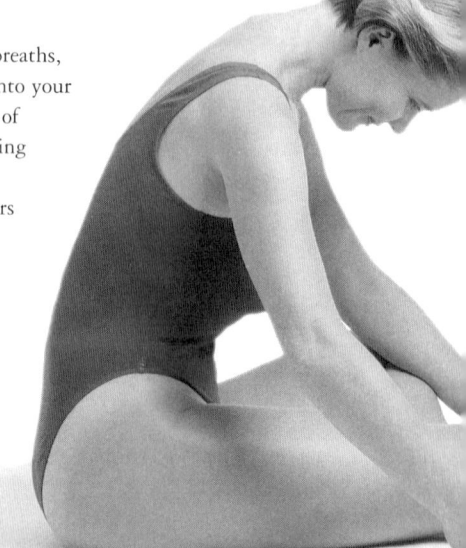

the foot. Your arms are resting on the floor, elbows stay soft and open.
▷ After twelve breaths, **zip up and hollow**, and slowly come back up into an upright position, rebuilding the spine vertebra by vertebra.

Repeat on the other side. Make sure that you stay central and do not twist over the leg.

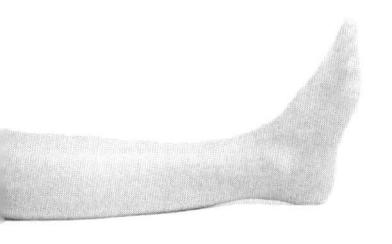

Side Rolls

Starting Position (called the Relaxation Position)
▷ Lie with your knees bent, feet hip-width apart and in parallel.

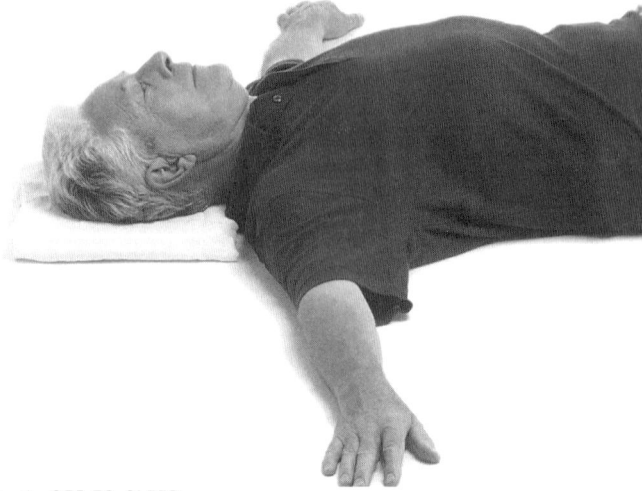

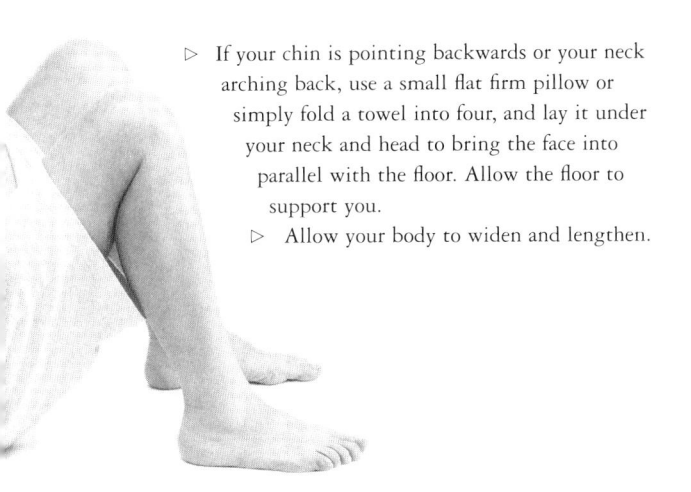

▷ If your chin is pointing backwards or your neck arching back, use a small flat firm pillow or simply fold a towel into four, and lay it under your neck and head to bring the face into parallel with the floor. Allow the floor to support you.

▷ Allow your body to widen and lengthen.

Side Rolls (continued)

Please note:
Please consult a practitioner before starting this exercise if you have a disc-related injury.

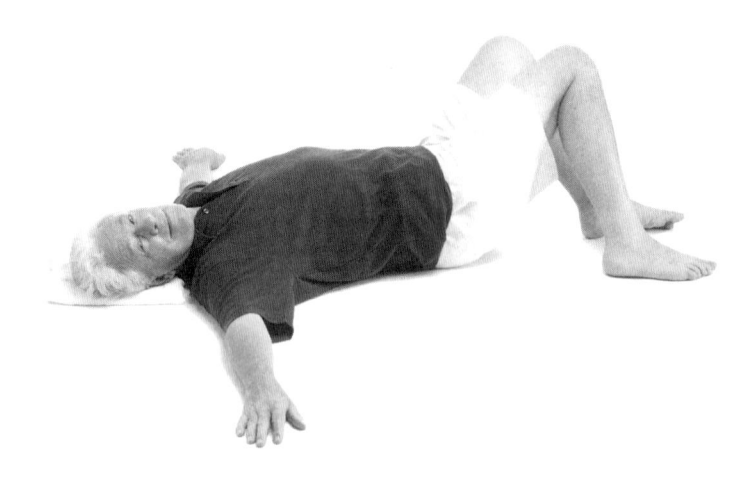

Action
- Place your arms palms down in a 'V' shape alongside your body.
- Breathe in to prepare.
- Breathe out, **zip up and hollow navel to spine**, roll your head in one direction, your knees in the other. Only roll a little way to start with – you can go further each time if it is comfortable. Keep your opposite shoulder down on the floor.
- Breathe in, still **zipping up and hollowing**.
- Breathe out, use your strong centre to bring the knees back to starting position, the head as well.

Repeat eight times in each direction. Think of rolling each part of your back off the floor in sequence and then returning the back of the ribcage, waist, small of your back, buttock to the floor.

Adductor Openings

Action

▷ Adopt the Relaxation Position, as on page 20.
▷ Breathe in wide and full to prepare.
▷ Breathe out, **zip up and hollow**, and bring one knee at a time on to your chest.
▷ Breathing normally now, place one hand under each knee and allow the legs to slowly open. This will stretch you inner thighs. Hold this position for two minutes, do not allow your back to arch.
▷ After two minutes, slowly close the legs and return feet one by one to the floor, while **zipping up and hollowing** navel to spine.

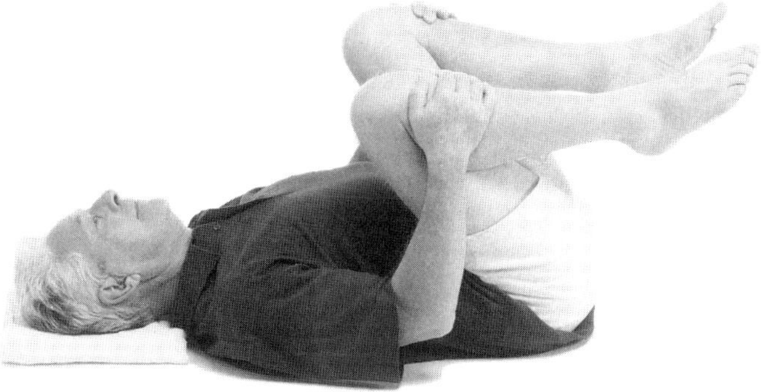

Shoulder Circles

Starting Position
This starting position comprises excellent directions for standing well throughout the day.

▷ Stand with your feet hip-width apart and in parallel, your weight evenly balanced on both feet.
▷ Check that you are not rolling your feet in or out.
▷ Soft knees.
▷ Find your neutral pelvis position but keep the tailbone lengthening down.
▷ **Zip up and hollow**.
▷ Lengthen up through the top of your head
▷ Shoulders widening.
▷ Arms relaxing.

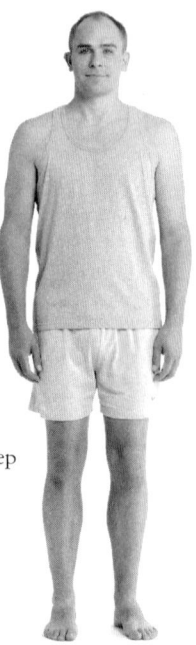

Action
▷ Breathe in and lengthen up through the spine.
▷ Breathe out, **zip up and hollow**. Then breathing normally, imagine that you have pencils attached to your shoulders and draw circles with them. Keep your back long, your abdomen hollow and your neck and head relaxed. Make the movement deep and slow.

Repeat ten times in each direction – it should feel like a wonderful shoulder massage!

Pelvic Roll Backs

Starting Position
- Sit on the floor, knees bent, feet parallel and hip-width apart.
- Hold your legs behind the thighs, just above the back of the knees.
- Keep your feet firmly planted on the floor with the weight evenly distributed.

Action
- Breathe in and lengthen up through the spine.
- Breathe out, **zip up and hollow**, now curl back onto

your tailbone. You are rounding your lower back and rotating the pelvis backwards. Do not come back too far to begin with. Keep hold of your thighs, the elbows stay open, the neck soft, your shoulder blades down into your back. Feet stay anchored.
▷ Breathe in, still **zipping up and hollowing** and uncurl the spine into an upright position again.

continued . . .

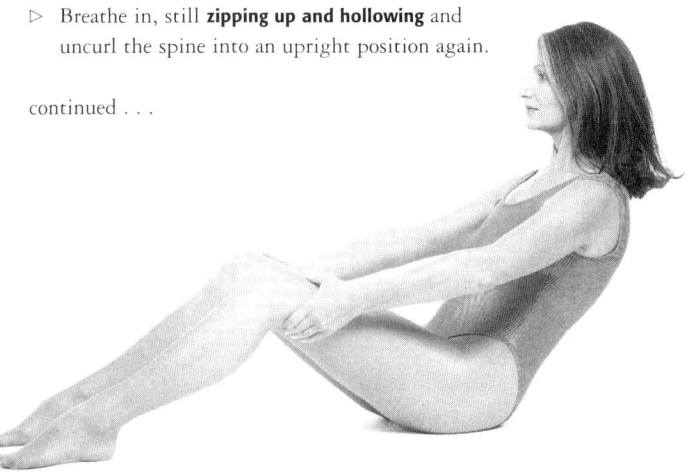

Pelvic Roll Backs (continued)

Action

You are now back in the Starting Position.

▷ Breathe out now, **zipping and hollowing** and, imagining that there is a cord attached to your breastbone, pulling forward and up, open the chest towards the ceiling and take your head back just a little to look at the top corner of the room where the wall meets the ceiling. *(See photo.) Don't let it drop back or take it back any further.* The neck stays gently lengthened.
▷ Breathe in and come to upright again.
▷ Repeat five times, checking that you do not roll your feet outwards.
▷ They should stay firmly planted into the floor.

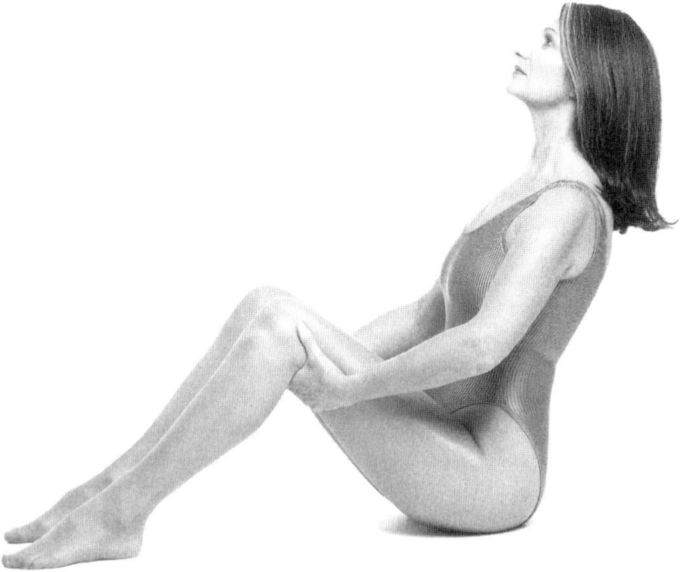

The Mexican Wave

Starting Position
▷ Sit on the floor with your knees bent, feet flat on the floor and in parallel. Alternatively, you can sit on a chair, whichever is the most comfortable.

Action
▷ Separate your toes, lifting them off the floor one at a time like a Mexican wave.
▷ Place them back on the floor one by one, beginning with the little toe and keeping them as widely spaced out as possible. Do not let the foot roll or your heels come off the floor.

Repeat five times on each foot. We never said it was easy! You may need to use your hands to help you move each toe separately.

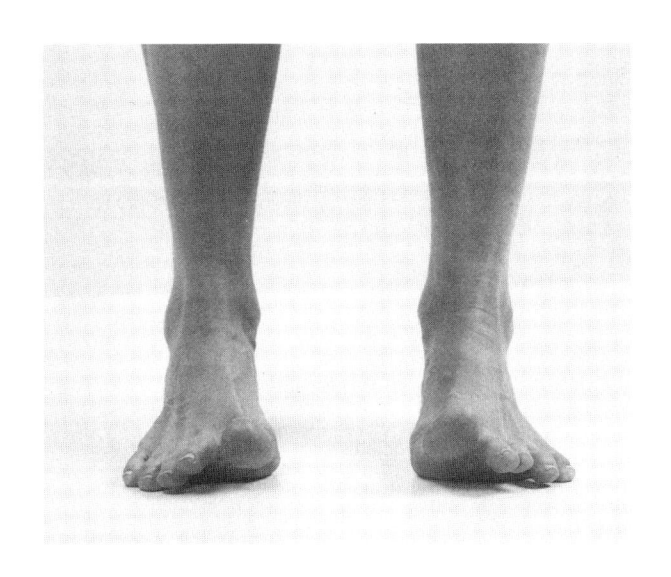

EXERCISES ▶ 33

Single Heel Kicks

Starting Position
You can either do this exercise with your head resting on folded hands or adopt the 'sphinx position' as shown in the photograph.

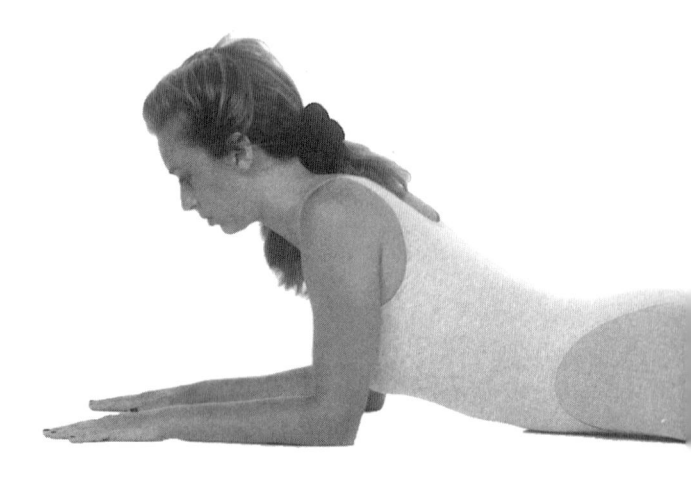

To adopt the 'sphinx position':

▷ Lie on your front. Place the hands on the floor just wider than shoulder-width apart.
▷ Breathe in and lengthen through the spine
▷ Breathe out, **zip up and hollow**, gently push down onto the forearms to raise the upper body off the floor. The elbows and shoulders stay down. Make sure that your neck remains long and you keep your pelvis and pubic bone on the floor. Throughout this exercise, you must keep zipped up and hollow! If you feel pinching in the lower back, come down to the alternative position, head resting on your folded hands.

The Single Heel Kicks (continued)

Action
Breathe normally throughout this exercise and keep **zipping up and hollowing**. The pelvis should stay quite still.

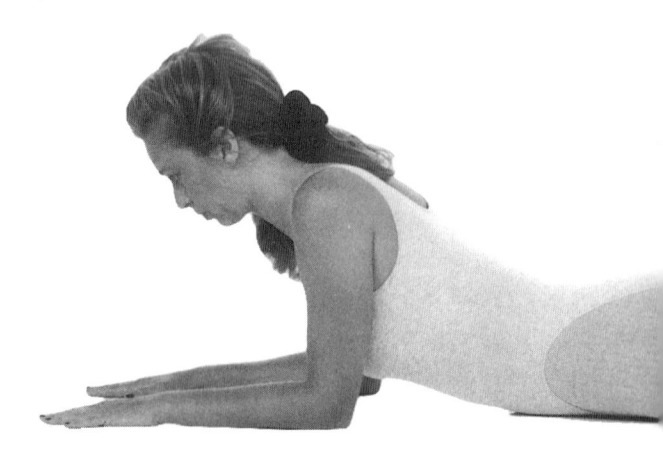

- ▷ Keep your legs slightly apart, and kick the right foot towards your buttocks, foot pointed.
- ▷ Release the foot slightly, then flex the foot and kick again, then slowly lower the leg.

Repeat ten times with each leg.

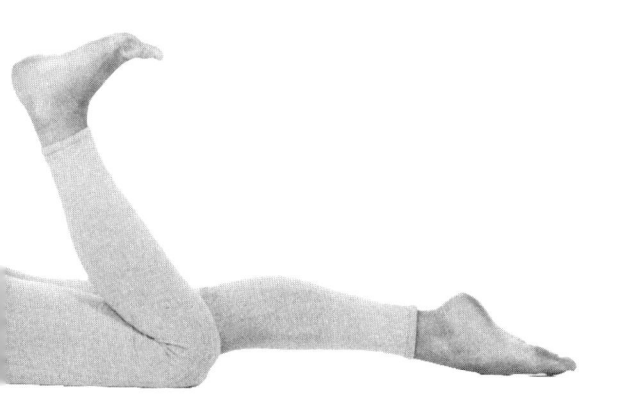

The Big Pillow Squeeze

Lie on your front. Place a small cushion between the tops of your thighs. Rest your forehead on your folded hands, open and relax the shoulders. Have your toes together and your heels apart.

Action
▷ Breathe in to prepare and lengthen through the spine.
▷ Breathe out, zip up from the pelvic floor and hollow the stomach. Imagine a fragile egg under your stomach that you do not want to crush.
▷ Breathe in and release.

▷ Breathe out, **zip up the pelvic floor and hollow the lower abdomen**. Now add tightening the buttocks, squeezing the inner thighs and the cushion and bring the heels together.
▷ Keep breathing normally and check that you are only working from the waist down. Hold for the count of five.

Repeat five times, keeping your feet on the floor, shoulders and neck relaxed.

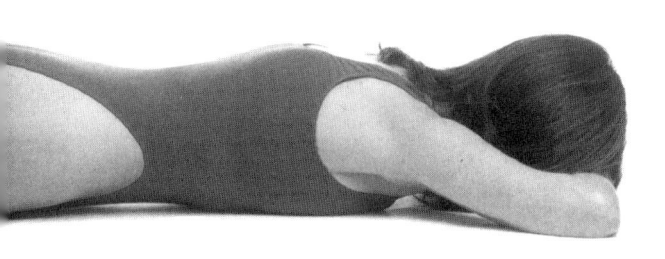

The Rest Position

If you have a knee injury, curl up on your side in a foetal position.

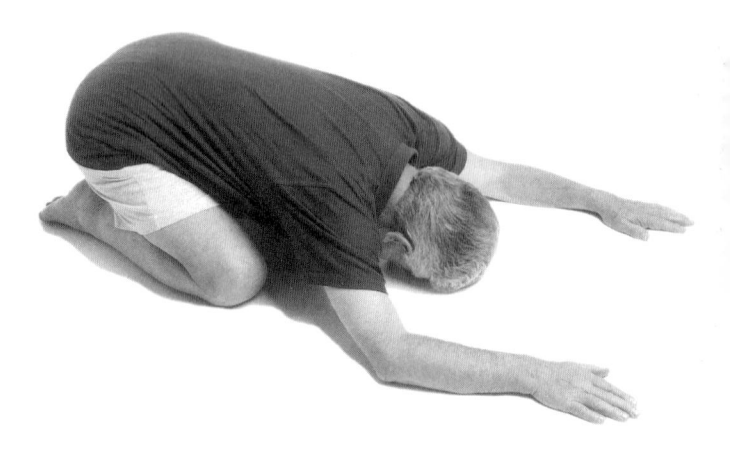

When you have finished the Big Pillow Squeeze, come up onto all fours, bring your feet together, but leave your knees apart and sit back onto your heels – not between them. Take eight breaths in this position, breathing deeply into the back of your ribcage.

To come out of the Rest Position – breathe out, **zip up and hollow** and rotate your pelvis backwards and, keeping your head and neck released, slowly start to uncurl, re-stacking the vertebra, one on top of the other, in order to come upright. Bring your head up last.

Circle Of Chalk

Please note:
If you have a shoulder or disc injury, please consult your practitioner before starting this exercise.

Starting Position
- ▷ Lie on your side with a pillow under your head – a bed pillow is perfect.
- ▷ Have your back in a straight line but curl your knees up to hip level at a 90-degree angle to your body – line all your bones up on top of each other.
- ▷ Extend your arms in front of you, in line with your shoulders, palms together.

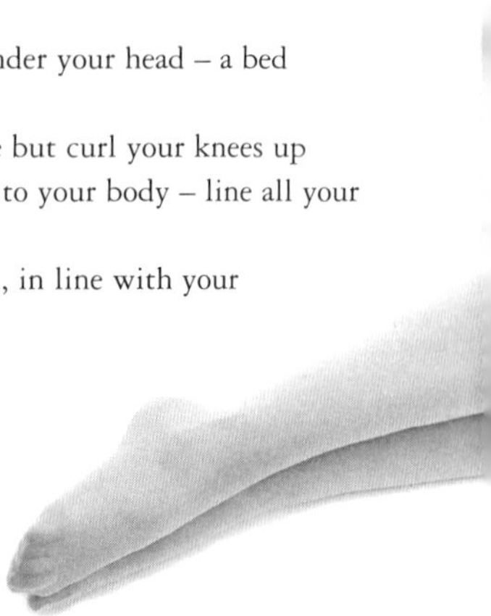

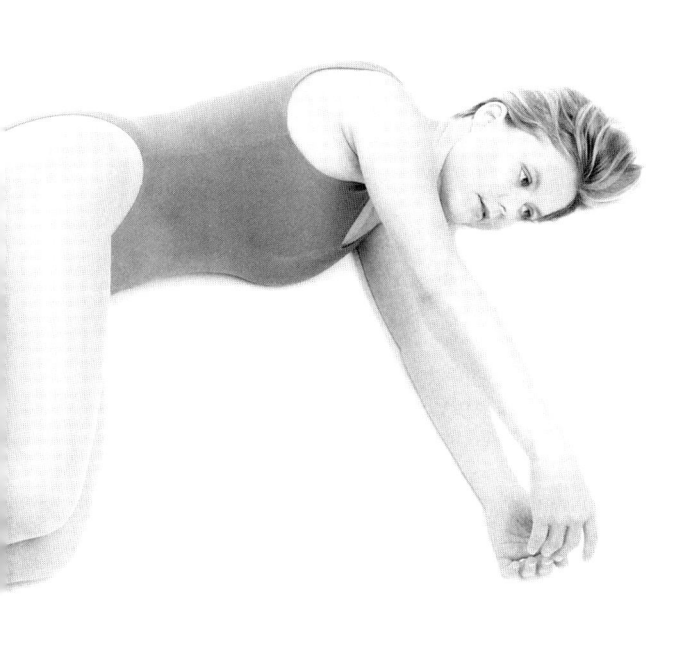

Circle of Chalk

Action
▷ Breathe in to prepare and lengthen through the spine.
▷ Breathe out, **zip up and hollow.** Imagining you have a piece of chalk in your hand, reach the top arm beyond the lower arm, taking your hand above you over your head. Allow your head to follow the movement of the shoulders. The knees stay together and the centre strong.
▷ Breathe normally now, reach your hand right around as if you are drawing a circle on the floor. It will pass behind you, down over your buttocks and back up to join the other hand.

Repeat five times on each side. The aim is to keep the hand in contact with the floor but, as that's difficult, please work within your comfort range.

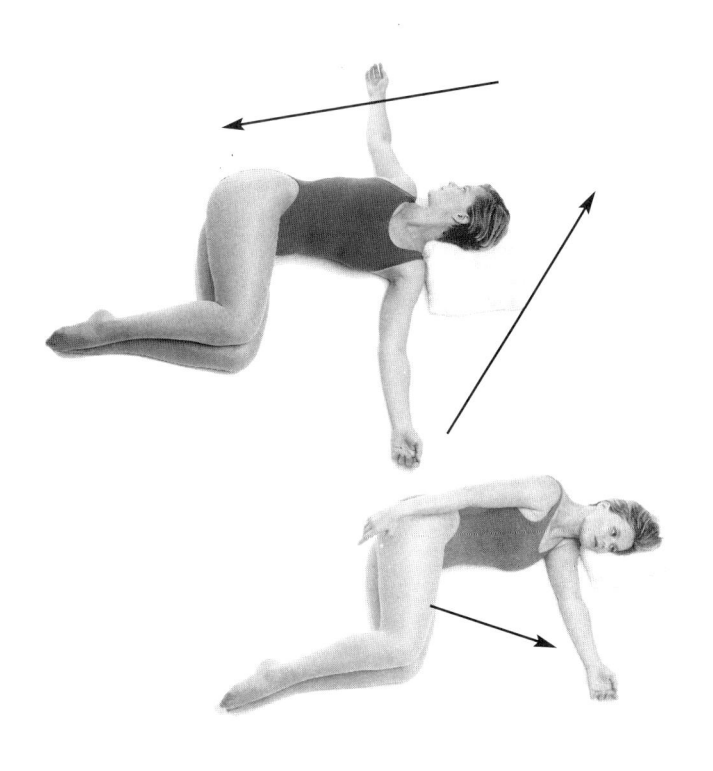

EXERCISES ▶ 45

Tense and Release – The Ultimate Relaxer!

May we suggest that you make a tape of the following instructions, or perhaps ask a friend to read them to you?

Adopt the Relaxation Position on page 20.

- Start by becoming aware of your feet, especially the soles and the toes. Squeeze the whole of your foot tightly during your next in-breath. When you exhale, let go of all the muscles in the foot. Repeat three times.
- Send your awareness into your calves. On your next in-breath squeeze the muscles very tightly to the bone and then let them go again during your out-breath. Repeat three times.
- Become aware of your thigh muscles, including the hamstrings at the back of your thighs. Tighten the muscles, squeeze as hard as you can – muscle to bone. Release again on your next out-breath. Repeat three times.

- Send your thoughts into your buttocks. Squeeze and release three times.
- Imagine your pelvis being a bony bowl, containing vital organs. Let your next out-breath soften the bones and, as a result, the bowl is widening, providing more space for everything contained inside.
- Send your awareness into your spine, from the tailbone all the way up into your skull. Release your spine into the floor.
- Let your attention focus on your arms. From the shoulder joint into the upper arm, into the elbow, reaching the forearm, travelling into the hand, all the way into the tips of your fingers. Repeat the squeezing and releasing as above.
- From the arms, let your mind travel into your neck and head. The next out-breath melts the tightness, smoothes the forehead and releases the jaw.

And so to bed . . .

These fantastic Pilates books are all available from your local bookshop, or by sending a cheque or postal order as detailed below.

Body Control – The Pilates Way 0 330 36945 8 £7.99 pb
The original best-selling manual taking Pilates out of the studio and into the home
Mind–Body Workout 0 330 36946 6 £12.99 pb
A fresh approach to exercise combining Pilates and the Alexander Technique

Pilates Through the Day
A series of mini-books to help your body make the most of every day
The Morning Energizer 0 330 37327 7 £2.99 pb
The Desk Reviver 0 330 37328 5 £2.99 pb
The Evening Relaxer 0 330 37329 3 £2.99 pb
Off to Sleep 0 330 37330 7 £2.99 pb

Pilates – The Way Forward 0 330 37081 2 £12.99 pb
Coming in April 1999, a whole new range of exercises to get you fit, keep you supple and safely work to remedy your body's problems

Book Services By Post, PO Box 29, Douglas, Isle of Man IM99 1BQ.
Credit card hotline 01624 675137. Postage and packing free.

For further information on books, videos, workshops, equipment and clothing, send an SAE to Body Control Pilates Ltd, PO Box 238, Tonbridge, Kent TN11 8ZL.
For a list of Pilates teachers and teacher training programmes, send an SAE to The Body Control Pilates Association, 17 Queensbury Mews West, South Kensington, London SW7 2DY.

Regular information updates appear on the Body Control Pilates website at www.bodycontrol.co.uk